AMAZING
STRENGTH
OF VEGETABLES AND FRUITS

TABLE OF CONTENT

CHAPTER ONE

WHY VITAMINS AND MINERALS ARE THE SOLUTION

We all wish we were more alert, had better abs, and could concentrate better. Similarly, we frequently find ourselves wishing that our skin or hair were better. We hope we could sleep better at night and that getting out of bed would be a little bit simpler (those last two things are connected, by the way!).

This has caused a number of companies to spring up that are all focused on improving the way we feel, seem, and function. We spend a lot of money on fitness classes, skincare products, as well as sleep aids. We test a variety of
Crazy stuff like wearing blue-blocking sunglasses all day or energy-healing crystals (which are just as effective as trying very hard!) to improve sleep (yeah, that's a thing!).

We try these things because we are desperate and looking for solutions. We are open to trying anything. Each time, we believe we're on the verge of finding the solution and realizing our full potential.

We are hoping that ONE of these things will offer the solution and make us feel AMAZING because we know we can accomplish it. However, very few of these tactics actually make a discernible difference.

The Issue? We complicate things too much. And a significant part of this is because of the
How much advertising is constantly bombarded onto us. Actually, improving
It’s all about the fundamentals when it comes to how you feel and look.

Think about your present diet and lifestyle, which are both highly likely. If you can relate to any of the following, raise your hand:

• You fail to consume your daily requirement of five fruits and vegetables.
• You consume a lot of prepared meals and processed foods.

• You only visit the gym three times a week or fewer, and you don’t particularly enjoy it.

The remaining time, I’m on the go

• You don’t get adequate rest.

• You experience chronic stress as a result of pressures at work, in your family, and financially.

• You spend a lot of your free time watching cartoons on the couch.

• You spend more than eight hours a day sitting at a computer screen, with a bent back, staring at a bright screen

• You seldom ever spend any time outside.

• You consume tainted tap water.

• You inhale air that is polluted with smog.

Although it paints a fairly depressing picture, many of us may relate to it. We never eat.
We don't get enough greens, we overeat sugary meals, and we are constantly worried. Then we question why we don't feel completely fine!

The reality Is that our modern lifestyles are plain dreadfully bad for our health, even if you answered most of these questions correctly.
This is true all the way down to the fact that the majority of us are too comfortable; as a result, our bodies have lost the ability to deal with stress or hardship because we have "adapted" to a cozy, domesticated lifestyle.

Take walking outside as an example. The majority of us simply don't do this frequently enough, which prevents us from receiving the crucial sunshine stimulus necessary to urge the body to generate vitamin D, which in turn controls things like hormone production, sleep, mood, and even appetite!

Our body loses some of its natural rhythm without that crucial input, which is referred to as "external zeitgebers" in the scientific literature, and some processes are halted.

But being in the cold also has a great advantage. Even when the sun isn't shining, being outside increases testosterone levels, boosts our immune systems, and even helps us become better at controlling our own body temperatures.

Is It any wonder that we constantly feel "stuffy" when we never exercise this body part?

Even going barefoot on the ground exercises the tiniest muscles in the foot, and our bodies yearn for activities like diving into the water and holding our breath to exercise our lungs and balance our carbon dioxide levels. We also don't give them it.

And as a result, our bodies are drastically deteriorating. Liken an overweight, spoiled pet dog to a wolf in the wild. Which is better for you?

That house dog is YOU. Plus a life that is incredibly demanding and sleep deprivation…

Starting With Vegetables And Fruits Are The Answer.

The answer is to start with fruits and vegetables. Why?

Well, it's all fine and healthily for me to advise you that you should exercise throughout the day, eat well, and go for lengthy swims in ice-cold water first thing in the morning.

The issue is that we don't have time for it, and because of our current state of maladaptation, our bodies couldn't manage it.

Even changing your diet requires a lot of work and can be extremely challenging. Eliminating all of the undesired processed foods, cutting back on overall calories, increasing fiber intake, and decreasing simple carbs are just a few of the challenges. Therefore, the greatest place to start is by resolving one of the most significant problems with contemporary life. Specifically, the absence of micronutrients.

Vitamins, minerals, amino acids, fatty acids, antioxidants, and other active food elements are examples of micronutrients, which our bodies utilize for a range of diverse functions.

We literally are what we consume, something many people are unaware of. You hear this a lot, but a lot of people think it's a metaphor. However, your body actually uses the nutrients it absorbs to rebuild your body after you eat food.

For instance, calcium and magnesium are used in the construction of your bones. These support the health of your teeth, nails, and connective tissue (ligaments and tendons). Collagen, which is present in bone broth and helps to improve skin, is one such substance that benefits connective tissues.

You would be the healthiest and most productive version of yourself if you could just increase the amount of fruit and vegetables in your diet. You could then have the motivation and energy to do the remaining tasks after that.

Even more fat can be burned by boosting your metabolism with fruits and veggies.

It's not difficult to increase your diet of fruits and vegetables, as we will see in the remaining chapters of this book. Making a few little, deliberate changes can drastically improve your health and wellbeing.

This book will also go over many additional fascinating and intricate ways that fruits can enhance your health and performance, some of which can completely change the way you feel and look.

You'll be able to cure any of your ailments by choosing the exact fruits and veggies you require.
Current illnesses, and you'll know just where to find them. Let's start now.

CHAPTER TWO

AN INTRODUCTION/ VISUAL GUIDE TO VITAMINS

Let's look more closely at the individual advantages of fruits and vegetables before moving on. Of course, checking at the vitamin content should be the first step.

You might be surprised to learn that vitamins were just discovered a century or so ago. Doctors were aware that some meals were beneficial for treating particular physical diseases prior to their official discovery, but they did not know why.

For instance, scientists discovered that eating a particular number of limes each day or drinking the juice prevented sailors from becoming scurvy, therefore the British Navy began carrying limes on board ships as early as 1975.

However, Casimir Funk, who was employed in the UK before moving to the United States in 1912, did not
The name "vitamines," which eventually became "vitamins," originated in the USA.
Since then, research on vitamins has advanced, and while the majority of us are familiar with the names of the most popular vitamins, we may not always be aware of their functions. Vitamins come in two different varieties. These are both water-soluble and fat-soluble vitamins.

The vitamins that the body can store are known as fat-soluble vitamins. This means that if you don't use all of the vitamins you ingest, your body can store them for use later on when you do.

The obvious benefit of fat soluble vitamins is that you are less likely to develop a shortage if your diet suddenly lacks one of these nutrients. The drawback of these vitamins is that if you take too much of one of them, your body won't be able to eliminate the excess and you risk developing a vitamin overdose.

Vitamins In Fat Form

The fat-soluble vitamins that are most well-known are vitamins A, D, E, and K.

Vitamin A keeps the mucous membranes smooth, supple, and moist, which helps to keep the skin moisturized. Additionally, it supports healthy bone growth, the preservation of reproductive system health, and healthy eyesight in low light. The foods whole milk, butter, eggs, and liver are sources of vitamin A. Carotenoids, a kind of vitamin A, are present in red, yellow, and dark green fruits and vegetables.

Calcium absorption by the body requires vitamin D. As a result, it, like calcium, contributes to strong teeth and bones. But both are important and complement one another. Foods that have been "fortified" with vitamin D include cereals and fat spreads. Since sunlight is the main source of vitamin D, it is frequently referred to as the "sunshine vitamin."

The reproductive system, muscles, and neurological system are all supported by vitamin E. It is an antioxidant as well. It is kept in the body because it is fat soluble and can help shield body cells from the impacts of free radicals, which can harm other cells.

Whole grains, almonds, wheat germ oil, and green leafy vegetables are all sources of vitamin E. Vitamin overdose is seen as harmful. Blood clotting is mostly caused by vitamin K. Without it, you would be at danger of bleeding to death whenever you cut yourself.

This vitamin also helps to build bone and kidney tissue. Liver, cheese, cereals, dark green leafy vegetables, and fruit are all sources of vitamin K. Additionally, it is produced in the intestines by good bacteria.

Vitamins that are water soluble cannot be stored by the body. Because of this, if you take too much of one of these vitamins, the extra is expelled in the urine. The benefit of water soluble vitamins is that an overdose is less likely to occur.

The drawback of these vitamins is that because they cannot be stored, you might need to consume higher doses. There is no reserve of these vitamins kept in your body, therefore if your diet is lacking in one of these vitamins even temporarily, you may experience vitamin deficiency symptoms.

Water-Soluble Vitamins

Vitamin C and the complete family of B vitamins are the two most well-known water-soluble vitamins. Ascorbic acid is another name for vitamin C. It supports the body's connective tissues, which make up the framework made up of muscle, fat, and bone.

It is an antioxidant, aids in the body's absorption of iron, and speeds up the healing of wounds by promoting the growth of new cells. Vitamin C also aids the body's immune system in fighting infections by protecting it.
Fruit, fruit juices, and vegetables are sources of vitamin C. The B group of vitamins includes thiamin (B1), riboflavin (B2), niacin (B3), pyridoxine (B6), and cyanocobalamin (B12). The main goal of this category of vitamins is to maintain the body working properly.

The body needs vitamin B1 to properly metabolize lipids, alcohol, and carbohydrates into energy. Unrefined cereals, seeds, and nuts, as well as lean pork, are sources of this vitamin.

B2 supports proper appetite regulation and aids in the body's utilization and digestion of proteins and carbs. Fish, poultry, pork, milk, and eggs are sources of B2.
Brewers yeast and dark leafy vegetables are both excellent sources of this vitamin.

B3 is necessary for healthy development and for allowing oxygen to reach bodily tissues. It is also in charge of preserving a normal appetite. Meat, fortified cereals, and bread are sources of vitamin B3.

B6 is in charge of drawing energy and nutrients from the food we eat. By reducing blood levels of excess homocysteine, it helps prevent heart disease. Soybeans, meat, nuts, eggs, whole grains, fish, lamb, poultry, and milk are all sources of B6.

Making healthy red blood cells is aided by B12. Additionally, it allows the body's nerve cells to communicate with one another, allowing us to hear, move, think, and perform other daily activities. In the small intestine of the body, bacteria produce it.

Although it is a water soluble vitamin, this one may be kept in the liver and is added to many meals, including cereals. Poultry, fish, milk, meat, and eggs are all sources of B12.

Eating a balanced diet is the greatest method to make sure you get enough of the water- and fat-soluble vitamins. You should seek medical assistance if you suspect that you may be vitamin deficient.

CHAPTER THREE: AN INTRODUCTION TO MINERALS AND OTHER WONDERFUL NUTRITION IN VEGETABLES AND FRUITS

INTRODUCTION TO MINERALS

Although both fruits and veggies are rich in both, fruits are often filled with vitamins, while vegetables are typically rich in minerals.

So, a nice place to start could be: What makes a vitamin different from a mineral?

Minerals are in contrast to vitamins, which are organic and so often extremely volatile (they can be destroyed by things like heat, air, and acid). In reality, a mineral can be a metal or a rock, which you might not typically consider to be essential components of who you are.

However, minerals are indeed essential to the human body's healthy operation. For instance, the body needs iron to form hemoglobin, which is a component of the red blood cells that carry oxygen throughout the body.

Without this procedure, the body would be unable to supply energy for the many essential processes that take place, including breathing, digestion, and more.

Minerals typically have a more essential role in the harder and more structurally important parts of the human body. Minerals, for instance, help to create ligaments, tendons, and bones.

However, minerals also contribute to conduction. After all, electricity powers the body, and keeping it charged properly is essential for the healthy operation of our muscles and brain.

Because the body cannot properly communicate with the muscles, an imbalance of sodium and potassium might result in cramping. Similar to how calcium is required to manage the charge in muscle cells, a lack of it might result in decreased strength.

Did you realize? The seed or stone can be used to distinguish between a fruit and a vegetable. They are absent from vegetables! Among the foods with unexpected classifications are tomatoes (a fruit), coconuts (a fruit), avocados (a fruit), and cucumbers (fruit).

Additional Crucial Micronutrients

Fruits and vegetables are a significant source of key nutrients A and B in addition to vitamins and minerals. Essential fatty acids and essential amino acids are the two essential nutrients.

Because certain ingredients cannot be manufactured by the body, they are referred to as "essential" and must be received from diet. The fact that 99.9% of us aren't getting them that way should perhaps also serve as a hint as to how serious a problem this is!

Now tell us what these nutrients do.

In a sense, amino acids are the components of proteins. We obtain a lot of them from meat, which our bodies subsequently disassemble into their component elements to rebuild our tissue. We are literally what we consume, as we saw at the beginning of this book!

For bodybuilders and athletes looking to gain muscle, amino acids and proteins in general are crucial.

According to research, athletes should consume 1 gram of protein for every 1lb of body weight. Other advantages of protein include the fact that it is considerably more difficult to turn into fat and that just digesting it actually burns calories!

As a result, a lot of people will work diligently to obtain sources of meat-based protein and will consume significant quantities of chicken in an effort to develop stronger muscles. This may become difficult labor! But they overlook the fact that protein may be found in both fruits and vegetables (though vegetables are slightly superior in this sense).

Think about more sources of protein than just the protein shake and chicken you consumed.
how much of the chicken's side dish broccoli is there.
The body uses amino acids for a variety of additional purposes, including the synthesis of neurotransmitters (brain chemicals), digestive enzymes, and much more. They are also capable of generating.

Finally, necessary fatty acids are found in fruits and vegetables. These are crucial fats that improve our ability to absorb other fruits and vegetables and provide a number of extra advantageous functions, such as improving brain function (the brain is largely composed of fat!).

One of the strongest essential fatty acids available, omega 3 provides an incredible array of advantages. Although we frequently associate omega 3 with fish, it can also be found in significant quantities in seaweed, hemp seeds, walnuts, kidney beans, soybean, and other foods.

CHAPTER FOUR

VEGETABLES AND FRUIT FOR ATHLETIC PERFORMANCE

Your thoughts likely immediately go to the traditional choices when considering a diet to help you gain muscle. You'll probably concentrate mostly on foods high in protein, such as chicken, fish, and eggs. Only meta and steamed rice should be included in an athlete's diet, right?

However, this is by no means the sole food that will help you gain muscle and perform better. In fact, having a balanced diet that includes a variety of various food groups is crucial for every type of athletic endeavor, including bodybuilding, sprinting, swimming, long-distance running, and others. You must be sure to eat your fruits and veggies, in particular.

Looking to improve your sports performance using supplements? You might be interested to know that eating fruits and veggies can actually be more beneficial for your health, cost considerably less, and have a ton of other fantastic advantages!

Here are some illustrations.

The best fruits and vegetables for enhancing athletic performance

Beets

For athletes of all types and for muscular growth, beets are by far one of the most crucial vegetables.

This is due to the fact that beets are one of the best meals in the world for increasing nitric oxide. Nitric oxide acts as a "vasodilator" in nature. This implies that it may lead to dilation (widening) of the blood vessels (veins and arteries), which will promote the movement of oxygen and nutrients throughout the body.

As a result, the muscles receive more nutrients to speed up recovery as well as more oxygen and energy during exercise. You may be able to lift heavier weights for more repetitions, run farther, and recover more quickly.

Potatoes

Although they are frequently portrayed as the evil guys, carbohydrates are crucial for gaining muscle and for physical exercise in general. Because they are low in calories, high in fiber, and high in vitamin C (which helps with recuperation), potatoes are a wonderful carbohydrate option. If you eat after working out, the energy will go straight to your muscles and not your waist.
Spinach

Spinach is a leafy vegetable that contains a lot of protein and a lot of phytoecdysteroids. These are completely different from anabolic steroids, however they could have a comparable impact.
- with some research indicating they are a viable choice for promoting testosterone and muscle growth.

Kale

The vegetable with the most calcium is kale. In fact, calcium is crucial for your exercises because it not only helps to strengthen your bones but also your connective tissue and your contractions, giving you greater explosive power when you exercise.

Given its high protein content and low calorie count, kale is currently quite popular. It's a shame that it's so expensive though!

Mushrooms

Although mushrooms aren't strictly considered fruits or vegetables, it's acceptable to include them because they can be purchased in the same aisle and are suitable for vegans. In addition to being a fantastic source of protein, mushrooms also have a number of other perks and health benefits. They contain a ton of minerals, help speed up workout recovery, and much more.

It can only be a matter of time until mushroom protein shakes become popular.
appearing in health food stores!

Mushrooms also have the unique feature of containing vitamin D. In reality
They are one of the few sources of vitamin D in the diet! (Oily fish is another.)

This is significant because vitamin D is thought to be a master hormone regulator and is involved in boosting the synthesis of testosterone, which is one of the key anabolic hormones involved in the development of lean muscle and fat-burning.

Furthermore, new research has revealed that vitamin D is far more effective than vitamin C for boosting immunity and warding off colds and flu. Every athlete is aware of how easily a cold can ruin their training schedule, which can mean the difference between success and failure.

Carrots

A significant source of vitamins A, C, and K, carrots are generally healthful. The lutein in them, which may aid to boost energy levels and improve the effectiveness of your very own mitochondria, is what's so fascinating about them.

Your cells' energy factories, your mitochondria, turn glucose into ATP (glucose being the sugar that comes from carbs, and ATP being the usable form of energy in your body). This basically indicates that you can run faster and burn more calories even when you're resting if you eat carrots and other lutein-rich foods.

One study discovered that when rats were given lutein—which requires a source of fat to ingest, like milk—they spontaneously started running large distances in their wheel and burned significantly more fat as a result.

Apples

Vitamin C, another essential vitamin for boosting the immune system and assisting athletes in consistently training longer and harder, is abundant in apples.

Additionally, vitamin C raises serotonin to help with mental recuperation, promotes muscular tissue regeneration, and when combined with zinc, even boosts the creation of both testosterone and nitric oxide.

In addition to all of this, apples are a very good source of fiber, which can aid with bowel motions, food absorption, blood pressure, and other things. A healthy microbiome can support a healthy immune system, a better mood, weight loss, and many other things. Fiber is essential to promoting a healthy microbiome.

CHAPTER FIVE: AMAZING SUPERFOODS FRUITS AND VEGETABLES FOR MOOD, ENERGY , BEAUTY AND MORE

AMAZING FRUITS VEGETABLES AND SEAFOODS

So you don't have much of an interest in losing weight? Possibly, you already are
Are you content with your size? The best to you!

You might not be an athlete. You might not be in particularly good health.

problems?

Look, everyone should eat fruits and veggies. Here are some more instances of fruits and vegetables with dramatically diverse health benefits to further emphasize the point.

Leafy Greens and Broccoli for Beauty and Pregnancy

Fruits and veggies can definitely help you look better. That's all especially in the case of something as basic as your common broccoli!

Compared to some of the other superfood fruits and vegetables on our list, broccoli may be a little less "strange." But don't be fooled; this dish is still very nutritious and ought to be consumed more frequently by everyone.

To begin with, broccoli is an excellent source of fiber and can once more aid in bettering your digestion, bowel movements, and many other things. However, broccoli also contains significant amounts of fiber, potassium, collagen, iron, calcium, and vitamins K and C.

Let's begin by exploring that collagen. We all require this, yet very few of us actually do. Collagen has been shown to help with reducing back pain, improving skin elasticity, strengthening the nails, preventing leaky gut syndrome, treating knee pain, and generally toughening up your tendons, ligaments, and bones. Collagen has also been shown to help with improving brain function and fending off Alzheimer's disease.

This explains why foods like bone broth are so extraordinarily healthy for us. Additionally, more recent evidence points to an even stronger justification for collagen's potential significance. Researchers now believe that historically, bone marrow from animal carcasses would have provided a large portion of human nutrition. The claim is that hunter-gatherers might have lacked the tools necessary to handle huge game. However, we were highly skilled at finding and pursuing our prey.

The likelihood is that we would have frequently followed antelopes and other animals to the spot where lions and tigers attacked and killed them. They would have then completely depleted those creatures.
their meat, leaving the skeleton in the wake. At that point, clever and resourceful humans would have appeared, used our tactile hands to crack apart the bones, and then consumed the nourishing collagen from within.

If this is the case, our species must have evolved in a setting where bone's various components were widely consumed. And now we are thrust into a world where we seldom ever receive these essential nutrients. If so, broccoli may have much greater health benefits than we originally thought!

pregnant women should consider increasing their intake of broccoli and other vegetables.
a variety of greens. That's because many salad leaves and broccoli are healthy options.
source of folate, which all new mothers are advised to consume.

Pregnant women who don't consume enough folate run a higher risk of having issues, therefore many of them turn to pregnancy vitamins to artificially enhance their intake.

The major benefits of obtaining more nutrients through your diet as opposed to supplements should be emphasized at this point. Although supplements can be beneficial, the word itself gives the game away. They are meant to complement your daily diet.

This means that rather than replacing your regular diet, they should be taken in addition to it. Because they are coupled with several other nutrients, lipids, fibers, and other components in your diet, nutrients from your diet are significantly more effective than those taken in tablet form.

Together, these enhance the essential ingredients' absorption, which increases their effectiveness. The important thing to remember is that because the human body evolved while being exposed to these foods, it is best suited to extract the nutritious value in this manner.

It is not intended to take in synthetic nutrients. For this reason, so many people advise against taking vitamin supplements on an empty stomach. They simply function better as foods.

Cayenne Pepper for Losing Weight
greater use of testosterone
Meanwhile, cayenne pepper is still another effective weapon in the fight against inflammation. Due to its anti-inflammatory properties, this substance, which gives food its fiery flavor, is frequently found in ointments and creams. Since it reduces the amount of the chemical "substance P" in nerve cells, it is also a common pain reliever. If you do have a condition like fibromyalgia or arthritis, substance P is a perfect addition to your diet because it both induces inflammation and the perception of pain.

Flavonoids and carotenoids are also abundant in cayenne. These are antioxidants that lessen the risk of cellular damage, thus reducing inflammation.
The advantages of cayenne pepper are numerous and amazing. It has been proven to be an efficient appetite suppressor, for example, so if you have trouble staying disciplined on a diet, you may start finding it a bit easier to do so and, perhaps, start losing weight.

Cayenne pepper also has the potential to enhance digestion. Here is vital since it helps you better absorb nutrients from your food and gives you more energy while also preventing discomfort. The advantages you already enjoy from the other superfoods on this list will then be amplified by a factor of 11.

Additionally, cayenne pepper has been demonstrated to increase
testosterone. It goes without saying that this is the hormone that most people refer to as the "male hormone" and which is to blame for both the male sex drive and many other characteristics that set men apart from women. Men who have more testosterone have better immune systems, stronger muscles, less fat storage, more aggression, better recovery, and other benefits.
Men who don't get enough testosterone will have depressive symptoms as well as low energy, a bad attitude, and a lack of sex desire. Additionally, they battle with muscle wasting and weight gain. On the other hand, males with high testosterone display the characteristics we identify with the traditional 'alpha male' in addition to having muscular and toned bodies.

Due to the various health risks and serious dangers associated with steroids and other medicines, so many men attempt to increase their natural testosterone levels.

The fact that testosterone levels in men are rising by 1% annually over the world is really concerning. Along with a number of other issues, this is partly caused by the use of feminine products and their effect on our water (certain plastics and our generally inactive lifestyles). However, nutrition also has a MAJOR impact. It's time to start eating more cayenne pepper and less manufactured food.

Elderberry as Anti-Inflammatory

Elderberries are berries that are loaded with nutrients. It is a fruit that is once more missing from many of our usual diets, therefore you should think about reinstating it.

The simple fact is that most of us consume the same handful of fruits and vegetables on a daily basis. However, by doing it this manner, we are assuring that we actually obtain a lot of nutrients while excluding some others. The most diverse diet—the one that offers the widest variety of fruits, vegetables, meats, herbs, and other foods—is the healthiest diet. So what benefits does elderberry offer?

Many historical cultures, like the Ancient Egyptians, have utilized elderberries as a supplement or medication since prehistoric times. These fruits are extraordinarily rich in flavonoids, particularly our buddies the anthocyanins, which are potent antioxidants like resveratrol.

Elderberries have also been demonstrated to support increased cytokine production. These are the molecules that serve as messengers in our bodies, which regulate the immune system. Anti-inflammatory cytokines aid in reducing inflammation, whereas pro-inflammatory cytokines aid in promoting it. It basically ensures that the body can appropriately manage its own reaction to viruses and diseases as well as aid in the healing of wounds and injuries, so all of this is quite significant.

Many of us mistakenly believe that inflammation is always negative, but in reality, it can help fight off infections before they have a chance to spread and promote healing by bringing more nutrients to the area that is hurt. The issue arises when this reaction deviates from normal.

It turns out that elderberry may be quite beneficial at preventing allergies for similar reasons!

Elderberries are also quite good in battling and eliminating microorganisms, which makes them helpful in treating infections, colds, and a variety of other issues. The tiny berries' powerful antiviral compounds, which have been demonstrated to actually 'deactivate' viruses, are what make them so intriguing.

These act by preventing the viruses from using their haemagglutinin spikes to penetrate cell membranes, which ultimately makes them nearly useless. As a result, they are excellent in both treating and avoiding issues like rhinitis.

Of course, berries also typically have the vitamin and mineral content that you would expect to find in them.

CHAPTER SIX

HOW ANTIOXIDANTS CAN LEAD TO LONGER LIVE

Our food naturally contains antioxidants, and they are also a crucial component of many supplements. Antioxidant vitamins, minerals, and a variety of Naka Herb supplements are very popular today because they are something of a buzzword.

Why is this happening, exactly? What are antioxidants exactly? Here, we'll take a brief look at how cells function, how cells die, and the significance of antioxidants.

The cell wall and the nucleus are the only components of our cells that are important to understand in this context. The component of the cell that naturally binds everything together and gives the cell its round shape is the cell wall, which is surrounded by mitochondria.

The nucleus, sometimes known as the "control center," is the location of the cell's nucleus, which is its center. The DNA, or "blueprint," that determines a cell's appearance, behavior, and placement among other significant cells in the body, is kept here.

However, there are also "free radicals" in our bodies, which is why antioxidant vitamins, minerals, and Naka Herb supplements are necessary. In essence, free radicals are chemicals that circulate throughout the body and harm cells. They are a byproduct of a variety of activities, such as breathing (oxygen is reactive and damages cells) and exposure to excessive amounts of direct sunlight (the UV waves in the sunlight are radioactive and can damage our cell walls too).

These free radicals then do a great deal of harm to the body, which is enough to eventually make our skin appear older. Even though the harm is initially minuscule, it can gradually accumulate to the point where it is visible to the human eye and also affects skin cells. Because of this, excessive sun exposure will initially make you seem good and tanned but will eventually make your skin look aged and leathery.

But on a more serious note, eventually these free radicals will penetrate all of the cell walls, which will mean that they enter the nucleus, which contains the DNA. If they get there, they may harm your genetic code, which leads to mutations that alter the expression of the cell and prevent it from performing its function.

Since cells divide to reproduce (a process known as mitosis), when a cell divides, it copies its DNA to the other half, resulting in two defective cells. Your immune system works to stop this, and buying herbs online can help, but it would be great if it could be avoided. Because these dying cells can eventually cause the failure of entire organs as they spread and turn into cancer.

By eliminating the free radicals immediately upon impact, antioxidant vitamins and minerals from fruits, vegetables, and even supplements will aid you in accomplishing this and preventing them from ever inflicting that damage. Then, these will delay the onset of visible aging and aid in cancer prevention—not bad!

CHAPTER SEVEN

HOW TO SUCCESSFULLY IMPROVE YOUR HEALTH USING FRUITS AND VEGETABLES

You should now have a clear understanding of the top reasons to make sure your diet includes enough fruits and veggies. These can improve your health in a variety of ways, and if you currently experience fatigue, irritability, sickness, or even depression, you probably lack one or more of these micronutrients. Given that the vast majority of individuals today DO have some form of deficit, this should not be shocking.

The second concern is the best method for gradually incorporating these fruits and vegetables. Do any negative aspects exist? How many specifically do you need? Can't you just swallow a vitamin tablet?

What Percentage of Fruits and Vegetables Do You Really Need?

You may have heard that you should try to eat five or more different fruits and vegetables every day. Many government agencies and health groups offer this broad guidance. This quantity has been raised to seven in some organizations. Although it is wise counsel, it is also arbitrary.

Why do I say that? Basically, that idea is not supported by anything!

The health benefits of fruits and vegetables are not innate. Despite being fruits and vegetables, they are not healthy for you. Instead, they are healthy FOR YOU DUE TO ALL THE IMPORTANT MICRONUTRIENTS THEY CONTAIN.

The best thing we can do for our health is to just obtain as many of those micronutrients as we can as they are needed in various amounts and kinds. The better for you is to eat more fruits and veggies. And when you acquire your nutrients from natural sources like these, it is very difficult to overdose.

And if a product is heavily processed, there's a good possibility it no longer contains many nutrients, even if the label on the package says it counts as "one of your five a day." It is almost certainly significantly lower in fiber, at the very least.

As a result, the advantages won't be as substantial as they would have been had you eaten that nutrient directly. Use common sense and try to consume as many whole, unprocessed fruits and veggies as you can wherever you can!

Too Many Fruits and Vegetables Can Be Dangerous

But eating too many fruits and vegetables might be harmful to your health. Or, to be a little more precise, it is rather simple to hurt yourself by eating too much fruit.

Fruit is full of sugar and has a high acid content, which explains this. It is particularly harmful to your teeth because of both of these factors. Serious dental issues are often the result of switching to diets that are exclusively focused on smoothie consumption.

Avoiding consuming excessive amounts of fruit juice or fruit smoothies is one way to address this. Focus on consuming vegetable smoothies instead, as they often have far less sugar in them.

The fact that fruits and vegetables still contain calories should be taken into account. This is particularly true for items like avocados, which are currently very popular. Avocados can still cause you to gain weight, even if they are wonderful for increasing testosterone (due to their beneficial saturated fat content) and are helpful for individuals attempting to avoid carbs.

Don't fall into the trap of believing that because fruits and vegetables are healthy, they can't help you gain weight.

The fact is that you must still keep track of and control your calorie intake if you want to prevent weight gain.

CHAPTER EIGHT

MAKING A FRUIT AND VEGETABLE-RICH DIET

You should increase your intake of fruits and vegetables, and as we've already seen, there are many specific foods that have benefits that are particularly noteworthy. You should also attempt to include a variety of specialized vitamins and minerals in your diet.

But how do you carry out that strategy? How do you go from having trouble getting your recommended five a day to being able to eat a wide variety of healthy ingredients with ease?

Because you shouldn't be taking a nap, which is another crucial realization.
a reductionist strategy of looking for each thing separately. When you do
if you do this, you'll discover that you wind up spending a lot of money while ultimately receiving little benefit.
There are a ton of fruits and veggies in this book that you can look for.
especially to get advantages for your health, immunity, inflammation, energy levels, and beauty. As a result, you can be persuaded to believe you can choose the advantages you wish. But this strategy is flawed.

You just cannot seek out each superfood separately when there are SO MANY of them, all of which provide some sort of great advantage. Here is

This is particularly true given that many of them won't mix, many won't be found in your neighborhood grocery, and some won't be edible for long. What then do you do in its place?

The Strategy: Variety is the Goal

To get the most diversity possible in your diet, rather than looking for specific varieties of fruits and vegetables, is considerably preferable. By doing this, you will include the broadest range of substances in your diet and so get the greatest variety of advantages.

Even if you ate only the healthiest superfood veggie, you wouldn't reap its full benefits because you would only be consuming enormous quantities of the same ingredients.

Even if you ate only the healthiest superfood veggie, you wouldn't reap its full benefits because you would only be consuming enormous quantities of the same ingredients.

Although apples aren't typically thought of as superfoods, they are just as spectacular as those more exotic concepts since they contain significant amounts of vitamin C, an antioxidant that increases testosterone, promotes the synthesis of nitric oxide, and creates serotonin.

Moreover, the variety of nutrients you receive will be significantly greater if you consume three different fruits and vegetables.

Studies have also shown that a varied diet is best for our microbiome, the good bacteria in our stomachs. Your gut health will be stronger the more variety you consume, which will lead to weight loss, more energy, improved mood, and other benefits.

Finally, by focusing only on "eating lots of fruits and veggies," you can simplify your diet improvement and make yourself more likely to keep to your resolution.

How To Increase Fruits & Vegetable Variety

So how can you broaden the selection? Here are some quick ideas to help you accomplish that without making your subsequent shopping excursion very stressful:

• Prepare a lot of Italian foods, stews, and hot pots. It's actually very simple to just throw a lot of fruits and veggies into a pot with some mince when making something like a bolognaise.

• Try grating foods like carrots to make this process even simpler (you won't need to
Use frozen foods like sweetcorn, peas, and mushrooms (which are easier to peel).

• Produce a lot of salads! Grab some salad leaves, add some sweet potatoes, cucumber slices, and a squeeze of lemon for a quick cold lunch. This can be served as a side dish to almost anything you make. You can acquire iron and folate from baby leaf spinach. Then simply switch up which leaf you use each time.

• Freeze! When doing this, prepare big quantities of food in a variety of separately portioned tupperwares, and then freeze them. Then, when it's time to eat, all you have to do is defrost each one individually.

• Blend smoothies! Simply throw a lot of fruits and/or vegetables in and press the blend button to make these. They also offer an enormous increase of wonderful advantages. Some of the happiest and most energized people I know regularly drink smoothies!

• Stock up on fruits and veggies. Fruits are frequently available for purchase at the counter in cafes and stores alike. Just buy the fruit that looks the most exotic, rather than a chocolate-based snack!

CHAPTER NINE

A MULTIVITAMIN SUPPLEMENT, WHAT ABOUT IT?

If the vitamins, minerals, and other vital micronutrients in fruits and vegetables are what make them so beneficial, then it makes sense to wonder how multivitamins compare.

A supplement that has a balance of many nutrients is called a multivitamin. Typically, one might be found that has a complex of the vitamins C, D, A, and B. For "healthy bones and hormone balance," multimineral supplements may also include Iron, Magnesium, Potassium, Calcium, and Zinc.

Do these goods compare favorably to the "genuine deal"?

No and yes.

One the one hand, you can absorb vitamins and gain from them. Although some people would claim otherwise, there are many compelling arguments to the contrary. Did you know, for example, that there are a number of items that are made to completely replace your diet? These include products like Soylent, which purports to provide every nutrient the body needs in the optimal balance.

Is it a wise decision? In no way! But right now, it's important to remember that users of this product live, and they're generally in good health. Because of this, we can say with certainty that multivitamins can also be absorbed.

There's a catch, though. A multivitamin is only going to be as effective as the person who devised it, which is the first of these catches. For instance, we observed with lutein and other fat-soluble vitamins. To be absorbed into the bloodstream, they require a supply of fat. If you obtain them from natural dietary sources, the source of fat is likely to be there. You never know if you'll get them with a vitamin supplement.

Numerous other vitamins and minerals also interact in a similar manner, facilitating easier absorption of the other. Similar to vitamins, different minerals absorb at various rates, hence they should ideally not be combined into a single solution.

Having said that, if the decision is between utilizing a supplement and not consuming those advantageous nutrients at all, the supplement is obviously preferable. In fact, a supplement might be a very practical and simple approach to obtain the nutrients you want.
Alternatively, it may serve as a "backup" to your diet.

CHAPTER TEN: CONCLUSION

STEP-BY-STEP GUIDE TO IMPROVE YOUR HEALTH

The guide comes to an end at that point. Now that you've read this, you need to have a much better understanding of the specific fruits and vegetables you should eat, their advantages, and how diversity is actually more important than anything else.

Likewise, you should now be aware of the most effective methods for including such fruits and vegetables in your diet as well as for averting any potential problems.

Given everything above, the following is your step-by-step guide to significantly improving your health and happiness by eating more fruits and vegetables:

• Have one smoothie to start your day, but limit yourself to one fruit smoothie.

• Don't limit yourself to eating only 5-7 fruits and veggies per day. Grab as many as you can to ensure a diverse mix.

• Make use of a supplement as "back up." This is particularly helpful when locating more esoteric and uncommon nutrients.

• But be sure to read the guidelines and conduct your own research. To facilitate absorption, you might want to consider timing and including a source of fat.

• Implement techniques to make including more fruits and vegetables in your diet as simple as you can.

• Steer clear of processed foods and "empty calories" by substituting salads and carrot sticks for items like chips and chocolate bars.

The program should be continued for 30 days. You should discover that you have more vigor, motivation, and improved health.

• Change other aspects of your lifestyle with this fresh vigor!

www.ingramcontent.com/pod-product-compliance
Lightning Source LLC
LaVergne TN
LVHW052104160826
845678LV00015B/3345